BUILDING THE ULTIMATE BODY:

Achieve Your Fitness Goals

GERARD CARROLL

Copyright Page

Copyright © 2023 by GERARD CARROLL

Disclaimer: The information contained in this book is for general informational purposes only. The author and publisher are not responsible for any actions taken based on the information provided in this book. Readers should consult professionals in the respective fields for advice and guidance specific to their circumstances.

Any websites or resources mentioned in this book are provided as a convenience and do not imply endorsement by the author or publisher. The author and publisher have no control over the content and availability of these external sites.

Every effort has been made to ensure the accuracy of the information presented in this book; however, errors and omissions may occur. The author and publisher disclaim any liability for any inaccuracies or omissions in this book.

Trademarks: All trademarks, service marks, product names, or company names mentioned in this book are the property of their respective owners and are used for identification purposes only. Use of these names, trademarks, and brands does not imply endorsement or affiliation.

TABLE OF CONTENTS

INTRODUCTION

Building the Ultimate Body: Achieve Your Fitness Goals is your reliable companion on the path to realizing your fitness aspirations. In a world brimming with information on fitness and the pursuit of the ultimate physique, it's easy to feel overwhelmed and lost in a sea of conflicting advice.

This book is your key to demystifying the complex science of getting your dream body while making the process as simple as possible. Together, we will explore all of the concepts, methods, and practises that will enable you to achieve the body you want without needless complications.

With the knowledge contained within these pages, you will be equipped to set realistic fitness goals, understand the workings of your body, make informed nutritional choices, engage in effective workouts, and sustain your progress over time. We'll break down the barriers of complex jargon, fad diets, and overwhelming exercise routines, focusing instead on a simple, evidence-based approach.

By the time you turn the last page, you will have not only developed the ideal body you've always dreamed of, but you will also have nurtured a lifelong commitment to health and wellness. Our journey will take you through the fundamental elements of fitness, from understanding the science behind it to the practical steps you can take in your daily life.

Your objectives are within reach, and we're here to guide you every step of the way. So buckle up and join us on this fascinating journey into the world of fitness as we uncover 'The Simple Science of Building the Ultimate Body'.

CHAPTER 1: WHY YOUR BODY MATTERS

Knowing why your body matters is essential to starting a journey to build the ideal body and effortlessly reaching your fitness goals. Your body is more than just a means of transportation through life; it's the center of your existence. It's the physical embodiment of who you are, the tool with which you experience the world, and the canvas on which your life is written.

1. Health and Well-Being: Taking care of your body is essential to living a long and fulfilling life. Your immune system, energy levels, and capacity to fend off diseases are all impacted by a well-maintained body. Our health revolves around your body.

2. Physical and Mental Performance: Your body is the vehicle that propels your daily activities. Its physical performance is essential to your everyday life, whether you're lifting weights, running, or simply getting out of bed in the morning. In addition, a healthy body has a direct impact on your mental performance, which includes your ability to focus, be creative, and make decisions.

3. Self-Image and Confidence: Your perception of your body has a big impact on your self-worth and confidence. Having a positive self-image can help you feel more confident and better about yourself. Having the ideal physique can make you feel proud of and confident in yourself.

4. Relationships and Social Interactions: Your body has an impact on how you relate to other people, how you conduct yourself, and how you participate in social activities. Having a positive body image can improve these relationships and social interactions.

5. Quality of Life: Your physical condition has a significant influence on your overall well-being. Maintaining your physical fitness is essential to an active and satisfying lifestyle since it enables you to travel, engage in a greater variety of activities, and appreciate life's small joys.

6. Personal Growth and Potential: Reaching physical fitness objectives involves commitment, self-control, and hard effort. By changing your body, you can access a larger pool of personal development and reach your greatest potential.

To put it simply, your body is the blank canvas on which you can paint the masterpiece of your life. It is a temple, and as such, it is something you should take care of and value. Recognising the significance of your body is the first step towards creating the ideal body and, by extension, changing your life. If you accept this fact, you'll be well on your way to living a longer, happier, and more fulfilled life.

The Science Of Building The Ultimate Body:
Let's examine the science behind building the ultimate body. In the pursuit of the ideal physique, one of the most important things is knowing the

science behind the process. It's not just about pumping iron or adhering to the newest diet fad; it's about making decisions based on the fundamentals of biology, physiology, and nutrition.

1. Muscle Growth and Strength: Building muscle is the foundation of body transformation. To properly build muscle, you need to understand the science of muscle hypertrophy, which is the process of inflicting microscopic damage to muscle fibers during exercise, followed by growth and repair, which results in increased strength and size. By knowing the mechanics of muscle growth, you can customize your workouts to achieve the best possible results.

2. Nutrition and Energy Balance: Reaching your fitness objectives depends on the energy balance principle. The science behind this is straightforward: you gain weight if you take in more calories than you burn off, and you lose weight if you take in fewer calories. However, it's not just about calories; the quality of those calories counts, as macronutrient ratios and nutrient timing are critical for both fat loss and muscle growth.

3. Cardiovascular Health: Understanding the science of heart rate zones, VO2 max, and aerobic capacity helps you create efficient cardio routines that improve your heart health and endurance. Cardio workouts have a significant impact on your cardiovascular system in addition to burning calories.

4. Hormones and Recovery: Understanding the scientific properties of hormones such as insulin, cortisol, and testosterone will help you maximize your exercise and diet for better outcomes. Hormones are the body's messengers and are essential for fat metabolism, muscle growth, and recovery.

5. Neurological Adaptations: The science of neurological adaptations describes how your body gradually gets more proficient at doing particular exercises, resulting in enhanced strength and performance. Your brain and nerve system are essential for muscular control and coordination.

6. Metabolism and Body Composition: Having a clear understanding of your metabolism and body composition is crucial. Knowing your body fat percentage and basal metabolic rate (BMR) can help you create transformational tactics and realistic targets.

7. Progressive Overload: This technique, which entails progressively raising the resistance or intensity of your workouts to continuously challenge your body and stimulate growth and adaptability, is the cornerstone of strength and muscle building research.

8. Recovery and Regeneration: You may not make as much progress as you would like to if you don't get enough sleep, rest, and a healthy diet to support your body's healing and growth.

The path to creating the ideal body is, at its core, a scientific one. Through exploring the nuances of nutrition, hormones, cardiovascular health, muscle growth, and other areas, you enable yourself to make well-informed decisions and customise your exercise regimen for optimal results. This scientific basis streamlines the process and increases your chances of effortlessly reaching your fitness objectives.

Chapter 2: SETTING YOUR FITNESS GOALS

The first step to achieving the ideal body is setting attainable fitness objectives. These serve as a road map, directing your efforts and inspiring you to stick with it. Here's how to create fitness goals that are both clear and attainable:

1. Be Specific: Rather than settling for a general objective such as "get in shape," specify your explicit goals. For example, "I want to lose 10 pounds," or "I aim to increase my bench press by 20 pounds."

2. Make Them Measurable: To monitor your progress, your goals should be measurable. You can gauge your success by using metrics like body weight, body fat percentage, or workout intensity.

3. Set Realistic Goals: While having lofty aspirations is admirable, it's equally important to have realistic goals. Take into account your current level of fitness, way of life, and availability of time. Unrealistic ambitions can cause disappointment and frustration.

4. Prioritize Your Long-Term and Short-Term targets: To help you stay motivated and track your progress, set both long-term targets (like reaching a certain body fat percentage) and short-term goals (like reaching weekly or monthly milestones).

5. Think About Your Motivation: What makes you want to reach these fitness objectives? Knowing your underlying reasons can help you stay motivated and focused. Your "why" matters, whether it's to improve your sports performance, your appearance, or your health.

6. Time-Bound Objectives: Give your goals a deadline. Establishing a deadline for your goals makes them feel more urgent and keeps you from putting them off.

7. Break Down Big Goals: If your end goal is high, divide it into smaller, more doable steps. For instance, if you want to run a marathon, start with a 5k, progress to a half marathon, and so on.

8. Monitor Your Progress: Keep a log of your exercises, dietary habits, and other pertinent information in a fitness notebook or app. Review your progress on a regular basis to make the required corrections and remain on course.

9. Remain Flexible: Because life is unpredictable, it's acceptable to make adjustments to your goals as necessary. The important thing is to remain dedicated to your advancement.

10. Seek Professional Advice: If you're new to exercising, you might want to speak with a qualified nutritionist or personal trainer. They can assist you in creating a customised strategy and helping you set realistic goals.

11. Appreciate Your Successes: No matter how minor, acknowledge and appreciate your victories. Doing so will keep you motivated and involved in the process.

12. Maintain Accountability: Join fitness communities or hire a coach for additional accountability, or share your goals with a friend or family member who can encourage and hold you accountable.

If you have well-defined and attainable goals, you'll be better prepared to traverse the path to success. Keep in mind that creating and accomplishing fitness goals is a dynamic process; as you advance, your goals may vary. The important thing is to stay committed and enjoy the journey towards building the ultimate physique.

Defining Your Vision:

Your vision is the overarching, long-term aspiration that motivates you to dedicate yourself to creating the ideal body. It is the clear mental image of what you wish to accomplish in the areas of fitness and well-being. Here are some tips for effectively defining your vision before you start your fitness journey and set specific goals:

1. Think About Your Why: Your "why" is the central idea of your vision. Start by asking yourself why you want a stronger, healthier physique. Is it to increase your self-worth, improve your athletic performance, or improve your general well-being?

2. Visualize the End Result: To assist make your vision more concrete and inspiring, close your eyes and picture yourself having reached your ultimate fitness goals. What does your body look like? How do you feel? What are you capable of that you couldn't do before?

3. Be Specific: Even though your goal is wide, it should still be specific. Rather than just saying that you want to "get fit," define what "fit" means to you. Maybe it's the ability to easily do a particular activity, run a marathon, or have a certain body fat percentage.

4. Align with Your Values: Make sure your vision is in line with your basic beliefs and values. If your fitness objectives are in line with your values, you'll be more likely to stick with it and feel fulfilled along the way.

5. Examine Long-Term Effects: Imagine how your long-term goals for the ideal body would improve your relationships, general well-being, and health. A long-term goal with positive effects can be a strong incentive.

6. Establish Milestones: Although your vision is a long-term objective, divide it into manageable chunks that you can celebrate along the way. Milestones provide you a sense of accomplishment and motivation.

7. Write It Down: Put your vision into words. You can use a vision board with words and images that symbolize your goals, or you can write it down in a diary. Having a tangible representation of your vision can help you remember it every day.

8. Remain Open to Adaptation: As you advance in your fitness journey, your goals may change. Remain open to modifying them in light of fresh knowledge and realizations. Adaptation is a sign of development and a flexible strategy for reaching your ideal physique.

9. Share Your Vision: Talk about your vision with a friend, member of your family, or a group that supports you. Sharing your vision can help to motivate you, hold you accountable, and even offer insightful counsel.

10. Remain Committed: Although your vision will inspire you, it is your dedication that will push you to consistently take action. Remain committed to the everyday activities necessary to get you one step closer to your ideal body.

By taking the time to clearly define your vision, you lay the groundwork for easily reaching your fitness goals. Your vision serves as a constant reminder of what's possible and can drive you towards building the ultimate body you desire. Your vision is the North Star that guides your fitness journey. It provides purpose, clarity, and motivation.

Setting Realistic Objectives:
Setting realistic targets is a crucial next step after defining your long-term vision for constructing the ideal body. Your objectives are the smaller, more manageable goals that will eventually bring you towards your vision. Here's how to set realistic objectives effectively:

1. Align with Your Vision: Make sure that your goals are in line with your long-term vision. They should be incremental steps that, upon completion, help you reach your ultimate fitness objective.

2. Make Them Specific: Rather than stating that you want to "lose weight," be more specific about how much weight you want to drop and when you want to achieve it.

3. Make Use of Measurable measurements: Your goals ought to be measurable in order for you to monitor your development. Whether it's weight reduction, height rise, or strength enhancements, pick measurements that enable you to gauge your progress.

4. Take Time Frames into Account: Give your goals a date and set deadlines for when you want to accomplish them. Setting deadlines for your goals makes them seem more urgent and keeps you on track.

5. Break It Down: If your long-term goal is very large, divide it up into smaller, more achievable

goals. For instance, if your long-term goal is to run a marathon, establish short-term goals like finishing a half marathon or a 5k.

6. Prioritize: Arrange your goals according to importance, starting with the most important tasks. Setting priorities for your goals enables you to make a progression that makes sense and is doable.

7. Remain Realistic: Take into account your present fitness level, lifestyle, and available resources. Be honest with yourself about what you can actually achieve within a certain timeframe. Setting unrealistic goals might cause dissatisfaction and demotivation.

8. Challenge Yourself: Despite the need of realism, your goals should still be difficult. Aim for an easy goal; this will encourage you to push yourself. Strike a balance between hard and attainable.

9. Make Them Actionable: Rather than saying "lose 10 pounds," an actionable aim could be "exercise four times a week and follow a balanced diet." Actionable objectives should centre on what you can control and the steps you need to take to get there.

10. Adapt as Needed: Because life is unpredictable and goals may need to be adjusted along the road, be adaptable and willing to modify as circumstances do.

11. Monitor and Assess Progress: To stay motivated and make the required modifications, monitor your progress on a regular basis and determine how close you are to reaching each goal.

Having attainable goals will help you stay motivated, track your progress, and eventually work towards achieving the ideal body you've always dreamed of. Setting realistic goals is the link that connects your long-term vision with your daily actions. It lets you break down your grand fitness goal into manageable steps and gives you a clear path to success.

Chapter 3 UNDERSTANDING YOUR BODY

One of the most important cornerstones in your quest for the ideal body is a thorough understanding of your own body. Because each person is different, you must be able to customize your fitness and health journey by understanding the subtleties of your body. Here are some tips for improving your understanding of your body:

1. Anatomy and Physiology: To understand how your body reacts to exercise, nutrition, and lifestyle choices, start by learning the fundamentals of human anatomy and physiology. You will get an understanding of how your muscles, bones, organs, and systems work.

2. Body Composition: Be aware of your body's proportions of fat, muscle, water, and other substances. Knowing your body's percentage of fat and lean muscle mass can tell you a lot about how healthy and fit you are right now.

3. Body Type and Genetics: Understand that your body's reaction to different stimuli is largely influenced by your genetic makeup. Certain individuals are born with a higher metabolism, while others have an easier time gaining muscle. Knowing your body type will help you create more reasonable goals for your fitness journey.

4. Hormones: Learn the fundamentals of how hormones affect your body. Your metabolism, muscular growth, and general well-being can all be affected by hormones such as insulin, cortisol, and testosterone. Understanding how hormones fluctuate can help you make better decisions about your diet and level of activity.

5. Energy Balance: Gain an understanding of the relationship between the number of calories you take in and the number of calories you burn off. This balance is essential to controlling your weight and body composition.

6. Physical Limitations and Potential: Evaluate your physical capabilities and limitations. Identify any past injuries or health issues that may have an impact on your fitness goals. Seek advice from medical specialists as necessary to make sure you're operating within safe bounds.

7. input Mechanisms: Pay attention to cues like soreness, weariness, and energy levels. These can help you tailor your training and recuperation plans. Your body gives input on how it reacts to exercise, nutrition, and rest.

8. Personal Preferences: Recognise your preferences and the kinds of activities you enjoy doing. This can help you create a fitness regimen that you'll be more likely to continue with. For example, if you love to cycle, include it in your plan; if you prefer yoga, find methods to incorporate that as well.

9. Progress Tracking: Keep a journal of your workouts, diet, and physical changes. This information will help you determine what is and isn't working for you. Track and analyse your progress on a regular basis.

10. Seek Advice from Experts: When in doubt, seek advice from nutritionists, fitness trainers, or medical professionals. They may offer professional understanding of your body and direction towards reaching your fitness objectives.

11. Pay Attention to Signs of Overtraining, Injury, or Stress: Your body communicates its requirements and limitations. Give it the attention and rest it needs to thrive.

Building the ultimate body is not just about the destination; it's about the journey of self-discovery and self-improvement. Knowing yourself better will help you tailor your fitness and health choices to achieve your goals. Understanding your body is an ongoing process that changes as you advance on your fitness journey.

Body Types And Genetics:
Understanding body types and genetics is crucial to building the ideal body because it can act as a compass in the confusing world of fitness and physique development. These factors also affect how your body reacts to certain lifestyle choices,

diet, and exercise regimens. Let's take a closer look at body types and genetics.

Body Types:
Three main body kinds, often called somatotypes, exist. Most people are a combination of these types, but one type usually predominates:

1. Ectomorph: Often labeled "hardgainers," ectomorphs are typically naturally thin with a narrow frame, a fast metabolism, and trouble adding both fat and muscle. They may also find it difficult to put on muscle and frequently have a "skinny" appearance.

2. Mesomorph: Mesomorphs, who have a naturally athletic physique with a higher proportion of muscular mass and lower body fat, are thought to be "genetically gifted." They may gain strength and muscle more readily and usually respond well to exercise.

3. Endomorph: Endomorphs typically have a strong, solid build and have a rounder or softer physique with a tendency to accumulate body fat. They may find it easy to acquire weight but may also find it difficult to remove fat.

Your fitness and nutrition plan can be customized based on your somatotype. For instance, an ectomorph may need a higher-calorie diet and emphasize strength training to gain muscle, while an endomorph may need to watch their calorie intake and give priority to cardio to reduce body fat.

GenetIcs:
The way your body reacts to fitness activities is largely determined by genetics as well. Here are some ways that genetics affect your fitness journey:

1. Muscle Fiber Composition: Genetics can affect your athletic ability as well as your potential for muscle growth and strength. Fast-twitch fibres are necessary for explosive movements and strength, while slow-twitch fibers are essential for endurance. Genetics can also determine the ratio of fast-twitch to slow-twitch muscle fibers.

2. Metabolism: Your basal metabolic rate (BMR), or how well your body burns calories at rest, is influenced by your genetic makeup. Some people have a naturally higher BMR, which makes it easier to maintain a lean physique, while others may have a slower metabolism, which makes it easier to gain weight.

3. Hormones: Important for muscular growth, fat metabolism, and general health, hormones like insulin and testosterone are influenced by your genetic makeup.

4. Injury Susceptibility: Genetics might affect your likelihood of developing specific injuries, such as ligament and joint issues, which can have an effect

on how active you are and what kind of training you choose.

Genetics can determine where you start, but it's important to understand that genes are not destiny. Regardless of your genetic makeup, you can make significant progress in your fitness journey with hard work, a well-designed fitness routine, and a balanced diet. Additionally, genetics do not take into account the enormous impact that consistency, dedication, and lifestyle choices have on your fitness journey.

In summary, knowing your body type and genetic makeup offers important information that can guide your decision-making regarding your fitness and health objectives. Knowing your distinctive features allows you to customise your training to reach your full potential and strive towards the ideal body that complements your personal qualities and desires.

Chapter 4 NUTRITIONS FOR SUCCESS

Nutrition is a key component in building the ultimate body. It's not just about feeding your hunger; your diet is the fuel that powers your workouts, supports recovery, and affects your body composition. Knowing the importance of nutrition is essential if you want to easily reach your fitness goals. Here's how to use nutrition as a foundation for success:

1. Balanced Diet: The foundation of your nutrition is a balanced diet that should contain a range of nutrients, such as vitamins, minerals, proteins, lipids, carbs, and fats. Each of these elements has a distinct effect on your fitness and overall health.

2. Caloric Intake: You must be aware of your caloric intake in order to control your weight and body composition. A caloric deficit causes weight loss, while a caloric surplus causes weight gain. Determine your daily caloric requirements depending on your activity level and goals.

3. Macronutrient Ratios: The way your diet distributes the three macronutrients (carbs, proteins, and fats) will have a big impact on your physique and performance. Your specific goals will determine the proper balance, but generally speaking, you should strive for a balanced intake of each macronutrient.

4. Protein: Depending on your activity level and goals, the recommended amount of protein to consume varies. Lean meats, seafood, dairy products, and plant-based foods are good sources of high-quality protein.

5. carbs: Including complex carbs from foods like whole grains, fruits, and vegetables in your diet will provide you with sustained energy. Your body uses carbohydrates as its main energy source, especially during activity.

6. Healthy Fats: Fats are essential for many body processes, so don't cut them out. Look for foods high in healthy fats, such avocados, nuts, seeds, and fatty fish.

7. Hydration: Drink enough water throughout the day, adjusting based on the climate and your level of activity. Maintaining energy levels, controlling body temperature, and enhancing exercise performance all depend on proper hydration.

8. Micronutrients: Make sure you eat a wide range of fruits and vegetables to acquire a variety of vitamins and minerals. These micronutrients are important for your general health and can affect how well you exercise.

9. Meal time: When it comes to maximizing outcomes, the time of your meals and snacks can have a significant impact on your energy levels, performance during your workouts, and

recuperation. Nutrition before and after your workouts can be especially crucial.

10. Supplementation: While the majority of your nutritional needs should be met by a balanced diet, some people may benefit from taking particular supplements, such as protein powder, vitamins, or minerals. Before beginning any supplementation, speak with a healthcare professional or nutritionist.

11. Portion Control: Be mindful of serving sizes to avoid overindulging. When necessary, estimate portion proportions with your hands or measuring cups.

12. Consistency: It's important to maintain consistency in your eating habits and in your nutrition plan. This will assist your body adjust and provide you long-lasting results.

13. Mindful Eating: You can avoid emotional or thoughtless eating by practicing mindfulness when it comes to what and how you eat. You can also choose healthier foods.

14. Individualization: Keep in mind that a person's nutritional demands are different from another's, so customize your diet to meet your specific dietary needs, goals, and tastes.

It takes more than just exercise to build the ideal body; you also need to fuel your body with the right nutrients to support your efforts. A carefully thought-out and well-balanced nutrition plan can make all the difference in the world, enabling you to effortlessly reach your fitness goals and keep your body in good, vibrant health.

The Role Of Diet In Fitness:

Your food is just as important as your training regimen when it comes to reaching your fitness objectives and developing the ideal body. The adage "you are what you eat" is extremely true when it comes to fitness. Let's take a deeper look at the diet's critical part in your fitness journey:

1. Energy Source: The foods you eat provide the energy (in the form of calories) your body needs for exercise, recovery, and general daily functioning. Your body needs energy to perform even the most basic functions, and this demand increases significantly when you work out.

2. Nutrient Supply: In addition to energy, the nutrients in your diet—such as protein for muscle building, carbs for energy, and lipids for a variety of body functions—are critical for muscle growth, repair, and general health.

3. Muscle Building and Repair: Specifically, protein is essential for both. Resistance training causes microscopic tears in your muscle fibres, which can be repaired and rebuilt into stronger, more defined muscles. A healthy diet that includes enough protein helps your body repair and grow these muscles.

4. Weight Management: Nutrition plays a major role in weight management, which is essential for reaching fitness goals. Your diet directly influences your body weight and composition. If you consume more calories than you burn, you will gain weight; if you create a calorie deficit, you will lose weight.

5. Recovery and Healing: An adequate diet helps speed up recovery and lower your chance of injury. After a hard workout, your body needs nutrients to repair damaged tissues and reduce inflammation.

6. Hydration: Maintaining optimal body temperature and exercise performance depend on proper hydration; dehydration can impair workout efficacy and cause decreased endurance.

7. Hormonal Balance: You can achieve optimal fitness outcomes by balancing your hormones through food, which includes insulin, which affects metabolism, and testosterone, which is essential for muscle building.

8. Mental and Emotional Well-Being: Eating meals high in nutrients will improve your mood, cognitive function, and general mental health, which will help you stay motivated and focused on your fitness path. Your diet also has a huge impact on your mental and emotional well-being.

9. Long-Term Health: What you eat has an impact on your health in the long run. Eating a balanced diet can boost immunity, avoid chronic illnesses,

and lengthen life, so you can reap the benefits of your fitness efforts for years to come.

10. Sustainability: The best diets are those that you can stick to in the long run. Extreme or crash diets are frequently temporary and can result in a cycle of weight gain and loss. Sustainable diets are ones that you can eat and stay on.

In order to make the most out of your diet in your fitness journey, concentrate on eating foods that are high in nutrients, making customized meal plans, and adhering to a consistent diet. See a registered dietitian or nutritionist for individualized advice, and keep in mind that diet plays a supportive role in fitness, providing you with the nourishment and support you need to reach your ultimate body-building goals.

Chapter 5 THE POWER OF EXERCISE

Exercise has a tremendous impact on your general health, well-being, and quality of life. Its transformative power goes far beyond physical appearance. Let's take a closer look at this amazing power of exercise:

1. Physical Health: Exercise has been associated with a lower risk of chronic diseases like heart disease, diabetes, and some types of cancer. It strengthens your muscles and bones, improves cardiovascular health, and increases flexibility and balance.

2. Weight Management: Exercise can assist maintain lean muscle mass while shedding excess fat, and it can help create a calorie deficit that aids in weight loss. Exercise is a powerful tool for managing body weight and body composition.

3. Mental Health: Regular physical activity can improve cognitive performance, promote self-esteem, and lower stress levels. It also releases endorphins, the body's natural mood boosters, which minimize symptoms of anxiety and sadness.

4. Energy and Vitality: Exercise, ironically, makes you feel more energized and capable of handling everyday duties with ease. This is because regular exercise builds endurance.

5. Sleep Quality: Getting enough sleep is crucial for healing and general health. Exercise can improve sleep patterns by assisting in falling asleep more quickly, staying asleep longer, and waking up feeling more rested.

6. Metabolism: Physical activity helps you maintain a healthy metabolic rate, which makes it simpler to control your weight and body composition. Exercise boosts metabolism, which affects how your body transforms food into energy.

7. Strength and Functional Fitness: Physical activity improves both strength and functional fitness, which makes daily tasks easier and less taxing. You'll be more capable of doing things like carrying groceries, climbing stairs, or engaging in leisure activities.

8. Cardiovascular Health: Cardiovascular workouts, such as jogging or cycling, improve the efficiency of your heart and circulation system. Exercise also lowers blood pressure, improves heart function, and lowers the risk of heart disease.

9. Longevity: Exercise can help you live a longer, more active, and healthier life. Research has repeatedly shown that regular exercise is linked to longer lifespans.

10. Pain Management: By strengthening the muscles that support and shield the afflicted areas,

exercise helps reduce chronic pain disorders including back pain and arthritis.

11. Immune System: Excessive exercise without sufficient recovery might lower immunity, so it's important to find a balance. Moderate exercise can strengthen your immune system, making you less prone to disease.

12. Social Connection: Activities that promote social connection and support, such as team sports, fitness courses, or group exercise, help people feel a part of the community.

13. Self-Confidence: Reaching fitness objectives through physical activity can increase self-worth. Reaching physical milestones and noticing positive changes in one's body can also increase self-confidence and self-esteem.

14. Healthy Habits: Investing in your physical health increases your likelihood of making wise decisions in other spheres of your life, like stress reduction and diet. Frequent exercise also serves as a springboard for other healthy habits.

15. Brain Health: Exercise can improve memory, focus, and creativity. It also has neuroprotective effects that lower the risk of dementia and cognitive decline.

Developing a regular exercise regimen is one of the most effective ways to achieve the ideal body and a vibrant, healthy, and fulfilling life. The benefits of exercise go far beyond the gym or the running track. They impact every element of your life, from your physical and mental health to your general quality of life.

Types Of Exercise:
Variety is not only the flavor of life, but it's also essential to a well-rounded fitness regimen. Including a range of activities in your fitness journey can help you develop a healthy, resilient, and strong body. Here are some popular workouts to try:

1. Exercises for the Heart:
- Running: Increasing endurance and burning calories, running is a traditional cardiovascular activity.
- Cycling: Cycling offers a low-impact, heart-pumping workout whether done outside or on a stationary cycle.
- Swimming: This is a great full-body exercise that improves cardiovascular health and is easy on the joints.
- Aerobics: To increase endurance, aerobic sessions provide a range of dance-inspired motions together with high-intensity workouts.

2. Exercise for Strength:
- Weightlifting: The foundation of developing strength and muscle is lifting weights, whether with machines, barbells, or dumbbells.

- Bodyweight Exercises: You may perform exercises like push-ups, pull-ups, and squats anywhere you have access to your own body weight as resistance.
- Resistance Bands: These adaptable bands are handy for on-the-go workouts and offer resistance for strength training.
- Functional Training: This method improves general strength and balance by emphasising exercises that resemble everyday tasks.

3. Adaptability and Movement:
- Yoga: By combining positions and awareness, yoga improves flexibility, balance, and mental health.
- Pilates: Through deliberate movements and breathing, Pilates places an emphasis on core strength and flexibility.
- Stretching: Consistent stretching exercises increase range of motion, lessen the chance of injury, and relieve tension in the muscles.

4. HIIT, or High-Intensity Interval Training:
HIIT workouts are a great way to burn fat and improve cardiovascular fitness because they alternate short bursts of intense exercise with rest intervals. They also save a lot of time.

5. Training on Circuits:
- Circuit workouts are effective and can be tailored for different fitness levels. They typically consist of a sequence of stations that include strength and aerobic exercises.

6. CrossFit:
- Known for its varied and demanding workouts, CrossFit combines Olympic weightlifting, functional movements, and high-intensity training.

7. Summer Camp:
- Military training served as the inspiration for boot camp sessions, which frequently combine cardio, strength, and agility training.

8. Group Exercise Courses:
Classes having a social element, such as Zumba, spinning, or kickboxing, provide fun, instructor-led exercises.

9. Sports for Recreation:
Playing sports like basketball, tennis, or soccer is an enjoyable method to increase your agility and level of fitness.

10. Mind-Body Exercises:
- Mind-body exercises, like Qi Gong, Tai Chi, or meditation, highlight the link between mental and physical health.

11. Targeted Exercises:
Certain exercises, such as bodybuilding for muscle growth or powerlifting for strength, are tailored to meet specific objectives.

12. Workouts at Home:
- Online training programmes, resistance bands, and bodyweight exercises can all be useful for at-home fitness regimens.

13. Adaptive Strength:
Exercises for functional fitness concentrate on strengthening the core, preventing injuries, and optimizing daily movements.

14. Outside Recreation:
Hiking, trail running, and kayaking are examples of physical and mental health-promoting activities.

15. Cross-Modal Exercises:
These incorporate a variety of exercise components, providing variation and a thorough approach to general wellness.

Finding exercises that fit your interests, goals, and lifestyle is essential to a successful fitness journey. By adding variety to your routine and keeping things interesting, you can push your body to new limits and develop the ultimate body that is strong, flexible, and full of life.

Creating Your Exercise Routine:
Whether your goal is to improve overall fitness, gain strength, or lose weight, creating a well-planned exercise routine is essential to reaching your fitness objectives and building the ultimate body. Here's how to create your exercise routine:

1. Make definite goals:
- Establish your fitness goals. Your aims will dictate the focus of your practise. Are they to improve flexibility, build muscle, boost endurance, or lose weight?

2. Examine Your Degree of Fitness:
- Be honest about your current level of fitness; if you're not experienced, begin with a beginner's programme to prevent overtraining and injury.

3. Decide How Often to Work Out:
- Figure out how many days a week you can dedicate to working out. Since consistency is key, choose a timetable that fits your schedule and provides enough time for recovery.

4. Pick Your Workout Styles:
- Choose the routines you wish to incorporate. To build a well-rounded programme, think about combining cardiovascular, strength, flexibility, and functional exercises.

5. Create a Weekly Timetable:
- Make time for your workouts every day of the week. For instance, you may set out particular days to work out for cardio, strength, and flexibility.

6. Determine the Length and Efficacy:
- Indicate how long and how hard each workout should last. You can incorporate shorter, high-intensity sessions or longer, moderate-intensity workouts, depending on your objectives.

7. Get Ready and Wind Down:
- Set aside time for warm-up and cool-down exercises, such as dynamic and static stretches, to help avoid injuries and speed up recovery.

8. Gradual Overload:
- Put the progressive overload principle into practise by progressively increasing the resistance, duration, or intensity of your exercises to encourage ongoing progress.

9. Don't Forget Rest Days:
- Remember to plan days for active recovery or rest. These are important to avoid overtraining and to give your body time to heal and adjust.

10. Adjust Your Schedule:
- In order to keep your workouts interesting and target different muscle groups, add diversity to them. You may try switching up existing exercises, adding new ones, or rearranging the sequence in which you perform them.

11. Pay Attention to Your Body:
- Listen to your body. If you experience discomfort, extreme exhaustion, or indications of overtraining, be prepared to modify your training plan or take additional days off.

12. Record and Monitor Developments:

- Track your progress with a workout notebook or fitness apps. Record your movements, weights, reps, and any other pertinent information. This will help you stay motivated and modify your regimen as necessary.

13. Look for Expert Advice:
- A fitness trainer or coach can help build a programme that is appropriate to your needs and goals if you are unclear of how to organize your workout regimen or would need personalized advice.

14. Review and Modify:
- As you get fitter and your goals change, periodically reevaluate and modify your workout regimen. What works for you today might not be appropriate later on.

15. Savor the Journey:
- Make sure your fitness regimen is sustainable and pleasurable. If you look forward to and love your workouts, you'll be more likely to stick with it.

Exercise routine creation is a dynamic process that should change as you progress in your fitness journey. You can design a workout plan that will help you reach your ideal body and improve your general health and energy levels by establishing clear goals, customizing your routine, and maintaining consistency.

Chapter 6 CARDIOVASCULAR HEALTH

Heart health, also known as cardiovascular health, is an essential aspect of total well-being and a key element in creating the ideal body. It includes the health and optimal operation of your heart and blood vessels, which are in charge of pumping blood throughout your body, providing oxygen and nutrients to cells, and eliminating waste. To enhance and preserve cardiovascular health, take into account the following tactics:

1. Aerobic Exercise: Include regular aerobic exercise in your regimen. You can improve your cardiovascular health by participating in sports like cycling, swimming, jogging, and brisk walking.

2. Interval Training: One effective technique to enhance cardiovascular health more quickly is High-Intensity Interval Training (HIIT), which consists of brief intervals of high-intensity exercise followed by rest intervals.

3. Lifestyle Decisions: Refrain from smoking and drink in moderation. Smoking poses a serious risk for cardiovascular disease, and consuming too much alcohol can harm your heart.

4. Nutrition: Minimize processed foods, saturated fats, and extra sodium. Instead, embrace a heart-healthy diet full of fruits, vegetables, whole grains, lean proteins, and healthy fats.

5. Stress Management: Practices like deep breathing, yoga, meditation, and finding time for relaxation can all help reduce chronic stress, which can be harmful to your heart.

6. Weight Management: Cardiovascular health depends on maintaining a healthy body weight through nutrition and exercise.

7. Schedule Regular Checkups: Keep an eye on your cholesterol, blood pressure, and general heart health by scheduling routine checkups.

8. Sufficient Sleep: Make sleep a priority because it gives your heart the necessary downtime and recuperation. Aim for 7-9 hours of good sleep per night.

9. Hydration: Maintaining proper hydration helps to maintain blood volume and blood pressure, which is important for your cardiovascular system.

10. Family History: Talk to your doctor about the history of cardiovascular disease in your family, as genetics can affect heart health.

A key component of your fitness journey is cardiovascular health. By making heart health a priority with regular aerobic exercise, heart-healthy eating, and heart-healthy living, you can fortify your cardiovascular system, lower your risk of heart-related problems, and live a longer, healthier life with the ideal body you've always wanted.

Effective Cardio Workouts:

Effective cardiovascular workouts raise your heart rate, test your endurance, and help you reach your fitness goals. Here are some well-liked and efficient cardio workouts to take into consideration. Cardiovascular workouts, often referred to as "cardio," are essential for building the ultimate body, improving cardiovascular health, and burning calories.

1. Jogging
- Whether you prefer to run outside or on a treadmill, running is a well-established cardiovascular activity that requires little equipment and is an effective approach to increase heart rate and endurance.

2. Biking:
- Whether you ride outside or on a stationary bike, biking is a low-impact cardiovascular exercise that can build muscle in your legs and help you burn calories.

3. Water Polo:
- Swimming strengthens your upper and lower body while offering a fantastic cardiovascular workout that is easy on the joints. It is a full-body cardiovascular exercise.

4. Leaping Rope
- Jumping rope is a low-complexity, high-impact cardio exercise. It's a great way to increase cardiovascular fitness, agility, and coordination.

5. High-intense interval training, or HIIT:
- High-intensity interval training (HIIT) is a time-efficient and highly effective way to burn calories and improve cardiovascular fitness. It consists of short bursts of intense activity followed by short recovery intervals.

6. Training on Circuits:
- Circuit workouts raise your heart rate and promote muscle growth by quickly switching between strength and aerobic routines.

7. Class Aerobics:
- Engaging aerobic programmes, such as Zumba, dance workouts, or step aerobics, are a great method to increase heart rate and enhance cardiovascular fitness.

8. Sculling:
- Rowing works your legs, core, and upper body for a complete workout; rowing machines provide a low-impact, full-body cardiovascular workout.

9. Exercise Elliptical:
- Elliptical trainers target the upper and lower bodies while offering a low-impact, gentle-on-the-joints cardiovascular workout.

10. Climbing stairs:
Stair climbing is a great technique to strengthen your legs and increase your heart rate, whether you do it on real steps or a stair climber machine.

11. Boxing kicks:
Kickboxing classes mix high-intensity cardio and martial arts to provide a fun and demanding full-body workout.

12. Trekking
- Hiking in the great outdoors is a great way to mix fitness and adventure because it not only provides cardiovascular exercise but also fosters a connection with nature.

13. Hurdling:
- Sprinting, which may be done on a track or in open places, is a great way to increase speed and cardiovascular fitness since it includes brief bursts of maximum exertion.

14. Group Athletics:
Playing team sports, such as basketball, tennis, or soccer, is a great way to get a social and aerobic workout in addition to adding a competitive element to your workouts.

15. CrossFit:
- CrossFit sessions frequently incorporate strength training with high-intensity cardiovascular exercises like rope jumping, box jumps, and sprints.

Try the following advice to increase the effectiveness of your cardio exercises:

- Use dynamic stretches to warm up your muscles and joints before working out.

Select an exercise regimen based on your fitness level and objectives.
- Increase the length and intensity of your workouts gradually to prevent overdoing it and getting hurt.
- Keep an eye on your heart rate to make sure it's within the desired range for cardiovascular advantages.
- Use variation to challenge various muscle groups and maintain an entertaining workout.

Aim to incorporate cardiovascular exercise many times a week into your fitness regimen to enhance your cardiovascular health, burn calories, and strive towards your perfect physique. Keep in mind that consistency is the key to an efficient cardio workout.

Chapter 7 STRENGTH TRAINING

Strength training—also known as resistance or weight training—involves lifting weights, using resistance bands, or performing bodyweight exercises to increase muscle, strength, and general fitness. The following is a summary of strength training's advantages and how it can help you develop the ultimate body and achieve a well-rounded, strong, and functional physique:

What Is Strength Training:
The main objective of strength training is to build muscular strength and endurance by forcing your muscles to work against resistance. Strength training is a type of exercise that focuses on resistance against a force, whether it be your own body weight, free weights, machines, or other forms of resistance.

Strength Training Benefits:
1. Increased Muscle Mass: Strength training causes muscle hypertrophy, which is an increase in muscle mass that improves your metabolism and physical attractiveness.

2. Increased Strength: Strength training, as the name suggests, dramatically increases your strength, which facilitates daily tasks and improves athletic performance.

3. Weight Management: Gaining lean muscle mass can help you lose fat and control your weight by raising your basal metabolic rate (BMR), which

allows you to burn more calories when you're at rest.

4. Bone Health: Strength exercise can lower the risk of osteoporosis and fractures by increasing bone density.

5. Injury Prevention: Your body is protected from harm during physical activities by having a robust musculoskeletal system and better joint stability.

6. Improved Functional Fitness: Strength training will help you become more capable of carrying out routine activities like bending, lifting, and carrying, which will make life easier.

7. Improved Posture: You can reduce or avoid back and neck pain by strengthening the muscles that support your spine and posture.

8. Metabolic Health: Strength training can lower the risk of type 2 diabetes, increase glucose metabolism, and improve insulin sensitivity.

9. Cardiovascular Health: When done at a greater intensity and with fewer rest intervals, certain strength training regimens can be beneficial to the cardiovascular system.

10. Mental Health: Frequent strength training has been linked to better mental health, including a decrease in anxiety and depressive symptoms.

Effective Strength Training Workouts:

1. Free Weights: A variety of workouts that target various muscle groups can be performed with dumbbells, barbells, and kettlebells.

2. Resistance Machines: These devices make it simpler to target and isolate muscles by offering guided actions for particular muscle groups.

3. Bodyweight Exercises: These equipment-free workouts are great for developing strength. Planks, squats, pull-ups, and push-ups are a few examples.

4. Circuit Training: A circuit-style workout can benefit the muscles and the heart by combining strength training with cardiovascular intervals.

5. Functional Training: By simulating real-world motions, functional exercises increase general strength and range of motion.

6. Progressive Overload: Gradually up the resistance, weight, or intensity of your workouts over time to continuously push your muscles.

7. Perfect Form: Keeping your form perfect is crucial to avoiding injuries and making sure your workouts are efficient.

Creating a Strength Training Routine:

When designing a programme for strength training, take into account the following:

- Split up your workouts so that you focus on the upper body, lower body, and core on various days.
For most muscle groups, aim for two to three days of strength training each week.
- Include complex exercises (such as squats, deadlifts, and bench presses) that target several muscle groups at once.
- Incorporate a range of workouts to prevent overuse injuries and challenge various muscle groups.
- Give yourself enough time to recover and rest in between sessions.

Strength training can help you achieve your ideal body and maintain long-term health and well-being because it is a flexible and adaptable type of exercise that can be done by people of all fitness levels. Strength training can help you gain muscle, improve your strength, or improve your overall fitness.

Chapter 8 FLEXIBILITY AND MOBILITY

Let's examine what flexibility and mobility are, their advantages, and how to enhance them. Flexibility and mobility are vital components of physical fitness that frequently receive less attention than strength and cardiovascular endurance. However, they are critical for building the ultimate body, preventing injuries, and maintaining overall well-being.

Comprehending Mobility and Flexibility:
In order to achieve a full range of motion in your joints, you must be able to extend and stretch your muscles and connective tissues (such as tendons and ligaments). Having good flexibility enables you to move your joints and muscles in a comfortable and unrestricted manner.

Conversely, mobility is the capacity of a joint to move actively within its range of motion. It is directly linked to joint health and muscle activation. Mobility is not just about flexibility but also about control over your movements.

Advantages of Mobility and Flexibility
1. Injury Prevention: A healthy range of motion enables your body to move and adjust to a variety of activities. It also helps lower your risk of strains, sprains, and overuse injuries.

2. Better Posture: Good posture lowers the chance of musculoskeletal problems like back pain since flexible and mobile muscles and joints support good posture.

3. Improved Athletic Performance: In order to improve agility, power, and coordination in sports and physical activities, athletes need to have more flexibility and mobility.

4. Pain Reduction: Pain or discomfort brought on by tense muscles or limited joint movement can be lessened with increased mobility.

5. Joint Health: Regular mobility exercises help you keep your joints healthy and functional. They also lower your chance of developing osteoarthritis and other degenerative diseases.

Methods for Increasing Mobility and Flexibility
1. Stretching: Make sure your regimen includes both static and active stretches. Static stretches help increase muscle length and flexibility, while dynamic stretches get your body ready for action.

2. Yoga and Pilates: These methods, which incorporate a variety of positions and exercises that focus on various muscle groups and joints, emphasize flexibility and mobility.

3. Foam Rolling: Using foam rollers to perform self-myofascial release can assist reduce muscular tension and increase range of motion.

4. Mobility Exercises: Engage in joint circles, controlled movements, and bodyweight exercises that improve mobility to actively move your joints through their whole range of motion.

5. Resistance Training: Use resistance training to enhance your strength and mobility. Good exercises to start with are lunges and squats.

6. Massage and bodywork: Expert massages or bodywork methods can relieve tense muscles and enhance range of motion and flexibility.

7. Consistency: Including consistency in your weekly or daily practise will help you gradually increase your range of motion and flexibility.

8. Warm-Up and Cool-Down: Dynamic stretches and mobility exercises should be performed before exercising. Static stretching should be performed afterward to aid in muscular relaxation.

9. Breathing and Relaxation: By reducing muscle tension, deep breathing and relaxation practises can facilitate stretching and enhance mobility.

10. Pay Attention to Your Body: Gradually increase the intensity and duration of your flexibility and mobility exercises. Respect your body's limits. Do not push yourself too hard, since this might result in injury.

Although they are sometimes disregarded, flexibility and mobility are essential for your fitness journey. By adding these components to your routine, you may improve your physical health in general, lower your risk of injury, and realise the full potential of your body in your pursuit of the ideal body.

Chapter 9 RECOVERY AND REST

It's easy to get caught up in the chase of the perfect body and peak physical health, concentrating only on exercise and nutrition to the detriment of another vital component of health: recovery and rest. Because proper recovery is just as important to muscle growth, injury prevention, and general health as exercise and diet, let's explore the importance of recovery and rest and how to incorporate it into your fitness journey.

The Value of Recovery:
1. Muscle Growth and mend: Muscles experience microtrauma throughout exercise, particularly strength training. Recovery enables these muscles to grow and mend, becoming more robust and resilient.

2. Injury Prevention: By allowing your body to recuperate and adjust, getting enough sleep lowers your chance of overuse injuries like sprains and strains.

3. Hormone Balance: Sleep, in particular, promotes the release of growth hormone and testosterone, which are important for muscle growth and repair. Recovery is essential for preserving hormonal balance.

4. Immune System Support: By boosting your immune system, rest and recuperation can lower your risk of sickness.

5. Mental Health: Getting enough sleep lowers stress and enhances mental health, which enhances mood and concentration.

Techniques for Successful Recovery
1. Sleep: Get seven to nine hours of good sleep every night. Sleep is crucial for healing because it is when your body heals and renews itself.

2. Nutrition: To support muscle regeneration and glycogen replacement, consume a balance of carbohydrates and protein after an exercise.

3. Hydration: Drinking enough water is crucial for healing since it helps the cells absorb nutrients and expel waste.

4. Active Recovery: By increasing blood flow and lowering muscle discomfort, low-impact, light exercises like walking or mild yoga help speed up the healing process.

5. Stretching: To improve flexibility and ease muscle tension, incorporate frequent stretching, both dynamic and static stretches.

6. Foam Rolling: Foam rolling, in conjunction with self-myofascial release, can aid in the release of muscular knots and enhance mobility.

7. Massage and bodywork: Skilled massages and bodywork methods can induce profound relaxation and alleviate tense muscles.

8. Rest Days: Based on your level of fitness, allot one to three rest days per week to give your body time to heal.

9. Listen to Your Body: If you notice symptoms of overtraining, such extreme exhaustion, poor performance, or persistent injuries, make necessary adjustments to your regimen or add additional rest.

Mental Healing
In addition to the physical element, mental healing should also be taken into account. The following are some techniques to support mental well-being:

1. Stress Management: Practice stress-relieving activities such as mindfulness, meditation, or relaxation methods.

2. Hobbies and Interests: To maintain mental and emotional equilibrium, pursue interests and hobbies outside of fitness.

3. Social Connection: To keep up a positive social life, stay in touch with your friends and family.

4. Time management: Plan your activities to make sure you have enough downtime and leisure.

When you prioritize recovery and rest in addition to your workouts and diet, you can better achieve your goals, maintain a healthy body, and lead a balanced, fulfilling life. Realize that optimal results are not only achieved through intense exercise and strict nutrition but also by giving your body and mind the time they need to heal, rejuvenate, and adapt.

Chapter 10 MONITORING YOUR PROGRESS

Monitoring your progress is an essential practise in your quest to reach your fitness goals and build the ultimate body. It gives you insightful information, keeps you motivated, and enables you to make well-informed changes to your fitness regimen. Here's how to do it well and why it's important:

The Significance of Progress Tracking
1. Motivation: Keeping track of your progress helps you stay accountable and motivated. Seeing improvements helps you stay committed to your fitness quest.

2. Determining Success: By keeping track of your accomplishments, you can acknowledge and appreciate your tiny and large accomplishments. This will give you more self-assurance and motivation to keep going.

3. Adaptability: It allows you to modify your exercise regimen in response to your progress. If you're not seeing the kind of results you'd like to, you can adjust to improve your exercises and address any inadequacies.

4. Goal Evaluation: Tracking your progress allows you to determine whether you're on pace to meet your fitness objectives, and you can make any required adjustments to your goals to make them more challenging or achievable.

5. Avoiding Plateaus: Fitness plateaus are normal. Tracking your progress enables you to recognise when you're hitting a wall and put tactics in place to get through it.

Efficient Techniques for Tracking Progress

1. Maintain a Workout Journal: Write down everything you do throughout your workouts, including the exercises, sets, repetitions, and weights you lift. This will show you just how much strength you are gaining.

2. Body measures: Track improvements with regular measures of important body metrics including weight, body fat percentage, and circumferences (waist, hips, biceps, etc.).

3. Pictures: Take progress shots in uniform lighting conditions and from different perspectives. You can see how your body has changed over time by comparing these images.

4. Fitness applications and Wearables: A plethora of applications and wearable gadgets can monitor your exercise routine, calories burned, and other fitness indicators. They can offer both historical data and real-time information.

5. Performance Metrics: Tracking increases in these metrics is an obvious indicator of progress. Examples of performance metrics to keep track of

are running times, distances covered, and personal bests during strength training.

6. Self-Assessment: Track your progress by evaluating how you feel both during and after workouts. Signs of improvement include increased endurance, less weariness, and less soreness afterward.

7. Body Composition Analysis: To determine the amount of body fat and lean muscular mass, think about utilizing body composition scales or DEXA scans.

8. Speak with a Fitness Professional: Getting advice from a fitness specialist or personal trainer will help you create a customized monitoring schedule and measure progress precisely.

Keep an Eye on Frequency
Your objectives and preferences will determine how often you track your progress. The following are some points to consider:
- Weekly Check-Ins: Weekly tracking can be beneficial for certain individuals, particularly those who are trying to lose weight or improve their running times.
- Monthly Assessments: Tracking changes in body composition and strength increases can be done with monthly measurements.
- Quarterly Assessments: Take into account quarterly evaluations for long-term objectives, as

they offer a more comprehensive view of development.
- Pay Attention to Your Body: Pay attention to how it feels. If you experience weariness or see alterations in your performance, it might be time for a review.

Modifying Your Exercise Programme
Utilize the information you've obtained from progress monitoring to guide your selections. If your development isn't what you had anticipated, take into account the following modifications:

1. Adjust Workouts: To keep your body challenged, adjust the amount, intensity, or workouts.

2. Dietary Modifications: Adapt your diet to your objectives, whether they are maintenance, cutting, or bulking.

3. Rest and Recovery: Since overtraining might obstruct improvement, make sure you're getting enough rest and recuperation.

4. Consult a Professional: Get guidance from a fitness expert if you're unclear about how to handle a plateau or progress issue.

It's important to keep in mind that progress is not always straight-line, and that you may encounter occasional setbacks. By tracking your progress and making necessary adjustments to your strategy, you can stay motivated and better prepared to achieve your fitness goals and develop the body of your dreams.

Chapter 11 STAYING MOTIVATED

Sustaining your motivation during your fitness journey, particularly if you're aiming to achieve the ideal body, can be difficult. You may experience periods of doubt or frustration, but there are techniques to keep you inspired and dedicated to your objectives. Here are some tips for maintaining your fitness motivation:

1. Make definite, well-defined goals:
Make a clear definition of your fitness objectives. Whether your goal is to run a marathon, grow muscle, lose weight, or reach a particular body fat percentage, having specific goals will give you something to strive for.

2. Segment Objectives:
Break down more ambitious objectives into more manageable checkpoints. Honour every victory, no matter how tiny. These checkpoints give you a sense of achievement and keep you motivated.

3. Determine "Why":
Determine the deeper motivations driving your fitness journey. Your "why" might be anything from better health to boosted self-esteem to becoming a role model for your kids. Whatever your personal motivation is, it will be powerful.

4. Imagine Your Success:

Visualize yourself reaching your fitness objectives. See yourself with the stronger, more toned body, or increased endurance you've always wanted. This will support your motivation and attention span.

5. Monitor Your Development:
Track your success using a workout journal, fitness app, or other tools; even minor improvements may be highly encouraging. Record changes in body dimensions, strength, weight, or other pertinent data.

6. Remain Steady:
Fitness requires consistency, so set up a regular workout routine and follow it. The more consistent you are, the faster you'll see results and the more driven you'll feel.

7. Vary Your Daily Schedule:
Adding variety to your workouts will help you stay motivated and avoid boredom. Try trying new exercises or exploring alternative fitness activities to keep things fresh.

8. Locate a Training Partner:
Exercise with a friend or partner can increase your enjoyment of fitness and serve as a kind of accountability; you will support and encourage one another along the way.

9. Join a Community for Fitness:

If you're looking for support, encouragement, and companionship, think about signing up for an online fitness community, class, or group.

10. Give Yourself a Treat:
Establish a system of rewards for yourself when you reach your fitness objectives. This may be a new exercise clothing, a treat, or anything else that makes you happy.

11. Engage a Trainer or Coach:
A fitness professional can help you reach your goals by offering advice, responsibility, and experience. Their support and understanding can increase your drive.

12. Make Self-Compassion a Practise:
It's OK to have bad days; what counts is how you pick yourself up afterward. Avoid self-criticism and treat yourself with kindness. Recognise that obstacles and failures are possible on your fitness journey.

13. See Opportunities in Setbacks:
Recognise obstacles as chances to develop, learn, and adapt when you have setbacks or plateaus. Overcoming obstacles can increase the satisfaction you derive from your eventual achievement.

14. Be Educated:
Continue your education in nutrition and fitness; the more you comprehend the ideas and science guiding

your efforts, the more driven you'll be to use them successfully.

15. Go Back to Your "Why":
Remind yourself on a regular basis why you began your fitness adventure. When your motivation starts to wane, go back to your "why" and fire it up again.

Recall that motivation fluctuates and that experiencing highs and lows is common. What matters is your capacity to persevere through times of low motivation and maintain your dedication to your objectives. You can keep up the motivation required to achieve the ideal body and live a better, more fit lifestyle by putting these techniques into practice and remembering why you are seeking fitness.

Getting Past a Plateau:
Fitness plateaus can be frustrating and are a common challenge. It's crucial to understand that plateaus are a normal part of the process if you've been making progress towards your goal of getting the ideal body and then all of a sudden your results stop. Nevertheless, with the appropriate tactics, they are surmountable. Here's how to overcome exercise regimen plateaus:

1. Review Your Objectives:
Start by reviewing your objectives for fitness. Plateaus can occasionally be caused by goals that

need to be adjusted. Do your objectives still fit your present needs and abilities? If necessary, reevaluate and redefine them.

2. Modify Your Schedule:

Your body's adjustment to a regular schedule is one of the most frequent causes of plateaus. Change things up by adding new exercises, adjusting the weights, modifying the format of your routine, or attempting an entirely new fitness activity. Change can inspire fresh development.

3. Increasing Stress:

The technique of progressively increasing your workout volume, weight, or intensity is known as progressive overload. If you've hit a plateau in your workouts, it might be time to up the weight, increase the number of sets or repetitions, or reduce the amount of time you spend resting.

4. Nutritional Modification:

Examine your eating patterns. Are you eating the proper ratio of nutrients to achieve your goals? As necessary, make adjustments to your meal time, macronutrient ratios, or calorie consumption. Having a healthy diet is crucial to overcoming plateaus.

5. Rest and Recuperation:

Make sure you're recovering and getting enough sleep. Overtraining may result in injuries and plateaus. Make sleep a priority, schedule rest days, and partake in active healing exercises like yoga or walking.

6. Speak with an Expert:
Think about getting advice from a certified dietician or fitness specialist. They can offer professional advice and create a customized plan to get you over obstacles.

7. Consistency and Mentality:
Mentally taxing plateaus can be. Remain upbeat and continue your routine with regularity. Perseverance might make the most impact during these trying times.

8. Periods of Deload:
A deliberate decrease in training volume and intensity is called a deload. By giving your body time to adjust to the stress of prior exercise, it can help with recovery and breaking through plateaus.

9. Track Your Development:
Keep a running tab on your development. Keep track of your diet, exercise routine, and emotional and physical well-being. You can spot patterns in your data and make the required corrections by analyzing it.

10. Set Temporary Objectives:
Establish more manageable, immediate goals in line with your long-term plans. Reaching these

intermediate goals will help you overcome plateaus and increase your motivation.

11. Think About Psychological Aspects:
Plateaus can be caused by stress, worry, and other psychological issues. Utilize mindfulness or meditation to reduce stress, and make sure your workouts are conducted with an optimistic outlook.

12. Have patience:
Overcoming a plateau may require some time. Have self-compassion and faith in the process. You will advance with persistent effort; plateaus are transitory.

13. Try It Out and Keep Track:
Try out a variety of tactics to see what suits you best. Certain food changes work better for certain people, while exercise routine changes are beneficial for others. Keep an eye on your progress and make any adjustments in light of your discoveries.

Recall that reaching a plateau is a normal part of the fitness journey and can be overcome. They may also present a chance for resilience building, self-improvement, and body knowledge acquisition. You may overcome plateaus and keep moving forward towards your ultimate fitness and body objectives by tackling them with adaptability, determination, and a positive outlook.

Chapter 12 BUILDING A LIFESTYLE

Achieving the ideal body and physical well-being requires more than just sticking to a rigid diet and exercise schedule for a certain amount of time. It all comes down to designing a balanced, sustainable lifestyle that promotes your long-term health. Here's how to create a long-lasting, active lifestyle that transcends fitness fads and shortcuts:

1. Establish Sustainable and Realistic Goals:
Set sustainable, attainable goals for your health and fitness. Steer clear of excessive diets and difficult-to-maintain exercise regimens. Prioritise long-term, progressive reforms.

2. Develop a Habit of Physical Activity:
Make exercise a part of your everyday routine. Make it a goal to be active most days of the week, whether it be by walking and using the stairs or by engaging in organized exercise.

3. Make Nutrition a Priority:
Adopt a wholesome, well-balanced dietary regimen. Provide your body with complete, unprocessed nutrients and design a long-term, sustainable eating schedule. This entails moderation in the

consumption of your favorite foods as opposed to severe dietary restrictions.

4. Rest well and stay hydrated:
Regular exercise and a well-balanced diet are crucial elements of a healthy lifestyle. To aid in your recuperation and general well-being, make sure you're getting adequate water and making rest a priority.

5. Resolve Stress:
Managing stress is essential to living a balanced lifestyle. Engage in mindfulness exercises, relaxation techniques, or stress-relieving hobbies. Stress can be detrimental to both your general health and fitness progress.

6. Accept Variety:
To keep things interesting, mix up your routine with different physical activities. To keep your interest and stave off boredom, try out various sports, outdoor activities, and fitness regimens.

7. Establish a Support Network:
Embrace a community of friends, family, or fellow fitness enthusiasts who are as dedicated to leading a healthy lifestyle as you are. You can stay responsible and motivated with the help of others.

8. Ongoing Education:

Keep yourself informed about health, nutrition, and fitness. Get up to date on the most recent findings and fashions so that you can choose a lifestyle that suits you.

9. Adopt a Positive Attitude:
Instead of concentrating on your mistakes, have an optimistic outlook and concentrate on the strides you have made. Your success can be greatly impacted by the way you think about your lifestyle.

10. Plan and Get Ready:
Planning ahead and being well-prepared can help make leading a healthy lifestyle easier. Plan your meals, set aside time for exercise, and give your health top priority.

11. Consult a Professional:
Take into consideration seeking advice from certified dietitians or fitness experts. They can provide personalized advice and guidance tailored to your goals and needs.

12. Adapt to Life Changes:
Recognize that life is dynamic, and there will be changes, such as career shifts, family obligations, or personal circumstances. Be flexible and adapt your lifestyle to accommodate these changes while maintaining your health focus.

13. Practice Consistency:

Consistency is the foundation of a healthy lifestyle. Staying committed to your habits, even on days when motivation wanes, is crucial for long-term success.

14. Reflect and Adjust:
Periodically analyze your lifestyle to assess what's working and what isn't. Adjust your routines and choices accordingly to stay on track.

15. Celebrate Small Wins:
Celebrate your victories, no matter how minor they may seem. Recognizing your efforts and triumphs can strengthen your commitment to a healthy lifestyle.

Building a healthy and balanced lifestyle is an ongoing journey. It's about making choices that support your health and fitness goals while allowing you to enjoy life to the fullest. By following these concepts and having a long-term perspective, you can establish a lifestyle that not only helps you construct the ultimate body but also promotes general well-being and happiness.

CONCLUSION

In conclusion, "Building the Ultimate Body: Achieve Your Fitness Goals with Ease" is a complete book that gives you the information and tactics to alter your body and achieve your fitness goals with greater ease. Throughout the book, we've studied the science of constructing the ultimate body, defining reasonable fitness goals, knowing your body, and crafting a balanced nutrition and exercise regimen.

We've gone into the important components of fitness, from cardiovascular health to strength training, flexibility, and mobility. We've also highlighted the significance of relaxation and recovery, evaluating your progress, and staying inspired along your trip.

Remember, building the ultimate body is not a one-size-fits-all procedure. It's a highly customized path that takes devotion, persistence, and the capacity to adjust to challenges and plateaus. With the insights and guidance provided in this book, you have the tools to make informed decisions, set and achieve your objectives, and sustain a lifelong commitment to your fitness and well-being.

In the search of your optimal body, constantly bear in mind that the journey is as vital as the destination. It's about not only the physical transformation but also the mental and emotional growth, and the enduring advantages that reach beyond beauty. By using the ideas contained in this book, you can go on a path of enhanced health, increased vitality, and a more confident, stronger, and healthier you. So, stay focused, keep motivated, and embrace the opportunity to improve your body and your life with ease.

www.ingramcontent.com/pod-product-compliance
Lightning Source LLC
Chambersburg PA
CBHW050846260726
48660CB00006B/2461